Testosterone-Building Therapy

Unlocking Vitality By Understanding The Foundations of Testosterone Enhancement.

Title:
Testosterone-Building Therapy

Subtitle

Unlocking Vitality By Understanding The Foundations of Testosterone Enhancement.

Copyright © 2023 by (Enola Cormier)

Printed in the United States of America.

ISBN: 9798872162827

TABLE OF CONTENT

INTRODUCTION

As hormones play a critical role in the intricate tapestry of human physiology, testosterone stands out as a quintessential player in the symphony of health and vigor. Hormones are responsible for orchestrating a variety of body activities. The purpose of this introduction is to lay the groundwork for our subsequent investigation into the field of testosterone-building therapy. We will delve into the essential aspects that highlight the significance of this therapy, as well as the delicate equilibrium of hormonal balance and the overarching objectives of this comprehensive guide.

The Importance of Testosterone

Testosterone is a steroid hormone that is largely generated in the testicles of males and, to a lesser extent, in the ovaries of females. It is commonly referred to as the "man hormone." Although it is typically associated with male qualities such as a deep voice, facial hair, and muscle bulk, its influence extends far beyond the surface attributes that are commonly associated with men. For both men and women, testosterone is involved in a wide range of physiological and psychological processes, and it plays a multidimensional function in both of these.

Muscle Development and Strength:

Testosterone is an important factor in muscle development and maintenance. It promotes protein synthesis, which is the process by which the body constructs and repairs muscle tissues. Adequate amounts of testosterone contribute to increased muscle mass, strength, and general physical performance.

Bone Health:

In addition to its role in maintaining muscle mass, testosterone is also an important factor in bone density. It helps prevent disorders such as osteoporosis and contributes to the development of cells that are responsible for bone formation. Researchers have shown a correlation between low testosterone levels and an increased risk of bone fractures as well as a decrease in bone mineral density.

Libido and Sexual Function:

One of the most important hormones for sexual health and function in both men and women is testosterone. The preservation of sexual tissues, as well as libido and sexual desire, are all affected by such factors. In males, it is essential for the creation of sperm, while in females, it has a role in maintaining the health of the reproductive organs.

Mood and Mental Well-Being:

There is a significant influence that testosterone has on both mood and cognitive performance. A happy perspective, mental clarity, and overall well-being are all connected with levels that are adequate with adequate levels. Contrarily, low testosterone levels have been associated with irritation, mood swings, and an increased risk of depression. These symptoms have been connected to the condition.

Metabolism and Body Composition:

Testosterone impacts metabolism and contributes to the regulation of fat distribution throughout the body. It contributes to the preservation of lean body mass and the enhancement of energy consumption, both of which are important. Testosterone levels can become unbalanced, which can lead to changes in body composition, including an increase in body fat.

Cardiovascular Health:

According to research, there is a correlation between testosterone levels and the health of the cardiovascular system. Adequate testosterone levels may have a protective effect on the cardiovascular system, assisting in the regulation of blood pressure and contributing to an overall improvement in the health of the heart.

Having an understanding of the complex network of processes that are controlled by testosterone highlights the crucial importance of testosterone in ensuring that one's health is at its best. Having an awareness of the far-reaching impacts of this hormone lays the groundwork for a more in-depth investigation into the hormonal equilibrium and the methods that may be utilized to maximize testosterone efficiency.

Understanding Hormonal Balance

The delicate balance known as hormonal balance is what keeps the endocrine system, which is made up of a network of glands that create and release hormones, operating properly. For general health, achieving and preserving hormonal balance is essential since hormones are chemical messengers that control several physiological functions. Hormonal balance in the context of testosterone refers to both the proper concentrations of this hormone and its harmonic interactions with other hormones.

The Endocrine System:

Hormones are produced and released by the pituitary, thyroid, adrenal, and gonad glands, among other glands that make up the endocrine system. These hormones impact the body by moving through the bloodstream.

Hormonal Feedback Mechanisms:

Balance is maintained by complex feedback systems within the endocrine system. The pituitary gland and hypothalamus are important organs for testosterone. Gonadotropin-releasing hormone (GnRH) is released by the hypothalamus, which causes the pituitary gland to release luteinizing hormone (LH) and follicle-stimulating hormone (FSH). The gonads then create testosterone as a result of these hormones.

Synergies and Interactions:

Hormones do not operate in isolation; their actions are frequently linked. For example, while testosterone and estrogen are frequently associated with certain genders, they are present in both men and women and maintaining the proper balance between them is critical. Imbalances can cause a variety of health problems, including reproductive and metabolic concerns.

External Influences on Hormonal Balance:

Age, stress, food, physical exercise, and environmental exposures can all have an impact on hormonal balance. Although testosterone levels naturally fall as people age, lifestyle variables and environmental pollutants can accelerate or offset this loss. Understanding these extrinsic factors is essential for creating successful hormonal optimization techniques.

Signs of Hormonal Imbalance:

Recognizing indicators of hormone imbalance is critical for preventative health care. Fatigue, decreased libido, muscle loss, weight gain, mood fluctuations, and altered sleep patterns are all symptoms of testosterone imbalance.

Recognizing these indicators necessitates additional inquiry and intervention to restore hormonal balance.

A thorough understanding of hormonal balance lays the framework for the investigation of specific testosterone-boosting techniques. Recognizing the interdependence of hormones and their impact on general well-being is critical for developing a comprehensive strategy for testosterone-building therapy.

Target Audience and Goals of the Book

Understanding the individual needs of the target audience is critical for effectively adapting information and recommendations. This book is intended for people who want to take charge of their hormonal health, with a specific emphasis on testosterone optimization. The intended audience consists of:

Men and Women Seeking Hormonal Balance:

Individuals experiencing symptoms of hormone imbalance, as well as those interested in maintaining and optimizing their hormonal health, will find this book useful. It addresses both men's and women's issues, acknowledging that hormonal health is a shared priority.

Athletes and Fitness Enthusiasts:

Athletes and fitness enthusiasts who want to improve their physical performance, muscle development, and recovery should read this book. Having optimal testosterone levels is critical for reaching fitness objectives and overall physical well-being.

Middle-Aged and Older Adults:

Because testosterone levels normally fall with age, middle-aged and older persons seeking knowledge on aging, vitality, and preventing age-related health conditions will benefit from the material offered.

Individuals Considering Hormone Replacement Therapy (HRT):

Individuals who are interested in hormone replacement therapy as a possible treatment for hormonal abnormalities are the target audience for this published work. To empower readers to make decisions based on accurate information, it offers insights into the various types of therapy that are available, as well as considerations, risks, and advantages.

These are the overarching objectives that this book aims to accomplish:

Educate and Empower:

The book's goal is to teach readers about the significance of testosterone, the factors that influence hormonal balance, and the role of lifestyle and nutrition in optimizing testosterone levels. Knowledge empowers readers to take an active role in their health management.

Provide Practical Strategies:

A primary goal is to provide realistic and evidence-based testosterone optimization solutions. The book presents a full toolkit for readers to adopt in their lives, ranging from nutrition and exercise to lifestyle changes and various therapeutic therapies.

Promote Holistic Health:

Because hormonal health is intertwined with other aspects of well-being, the book promotes a more holistic approach to health care. This study investigates how stress management, physical activity, nutrition, and sleep all interact with one another to attain and maintain hormonal balance.

Navigate Hormone Replacement Therapy (HRT):

The purpose of this book is to present a balanced perspective on the various available options, as well as potential benefits, dangers, and considerations for individuals who are contemplating or currently undergoing hormone replacement therapy. The purpose of this document is to act as a guide for making informed decisions in conjunction with healthcare experts.

CHAPTER 1: FUNDAMENTALS OF TESTOSTERONE

The hormone testosterone, which is frequently referred to as the principal male sex hormone, is an essential participant in the complex symphony that is human physiology. Its influence extends much beyond the conventional notions that have been held historically, and it encompasses a wide range of physiological activities that affect both men and women. This section conducts an in-depth investigation into the fundamentals of testosterone, including its description, functions, and the complex hormonal control and feedback processes that govern its synthesis.

What is Testosterone?

Testosterone is a member of the androgen hormone family, which is responsible for the development and maintenance of male traits. It is mostly generated in men's testicles, with lower amounts produced in women's ovaries and both genders' adrenal glands. In terms of structure, testosterone is a steroid hormone generated from cholesterol that is categorized as an anabolic steroid due to its role in tissue building.

Chemical Structure:

Testosterone is a steroid with a molecular structure consisting of 19 carbon atoms organized in four rings. $C_{19}H_{28}O_2$ is its chemical formula. Because of this structure, testosterone has the unique capacity to bind with specific cellular receptors and produce dramatic effects on numerous tissues and organs.

Synthesis and Production:

The endocrine system regulates the intricate process of testosterone production. It starts with the hypothalamic release of gonadotropin-releasing hormone (GnRH), which stimulates the pituitary gland to release luteinizing hormone (LH) and follicle-stimulating hormone (FSH) (FSH). LH, in particular, stimulates the testicular Leydig cells to make and release testosterone.

Circadian Rhythm:

The synthesis of testosterone has a circadian pattern, rising in the early morning hours and decreasing during the day. This natural fluctuation is necessary for hormonal balance and the efficient functioning of body processes.

Conversion to Other Hormones:

Other hormones, such as dihydrotestosterone (DHT) and estradiol, can be formed from testosterone (a form of estrogen). These transformations are conducted by enzymes such as 5-alpha reductase and aromatase. Each of these derivatives serves a specific physiological function and contributes to overall hormonal balance.

Functions and Roles in the Body

The effects of testosterone are felt throughout the body, where it plays an important part in the development, maintenance, and regulation of many physiological functions.

- Strength and Muscular Development: Increasing strength and muscle development is one of testosterone's main impacts. It helps in muscle growth and repair by encouraging the production of proteins in muscle tissues. Lean body mass preservation and improved athletic performance depend on this anabolic effect.

- Bone Health: Because testosterone promotes the growth of osteoblasts, the cells that make bones, bone health is largely dependent on testosterone. Sufficient testosterone levels lower the incidence of fractures and diseases like osteoporosis by maintaining bone strength and density.

- Libido and Sexual Function: In both men and women, testosterone has a complex relationship with sexual health and function. It affects sexual desire intensity, libido, and the general upkeep of sexual tissues. It is essential for sperm production and the healthy operation of the reproductive system in men.

- Mood and Cognitive Function: The effects of testosterone on mood and cognitive function are significant. Sufficient amounts are linked to mental clarity, optimism, and general wellbeing. Low testosterone levels have been linked in studies to irritation, mood fluctuations, and a higher chance of depression.

- Body composition and metabolism are influenced by testosterone, which also affects how energy is used and where body fat is distributed. Lean body mass is linked to optimal levels, whereas imbalances can lead to alterations in body composition, such as an increase in body fat.

- Cardiovascular Health: New research suggests a link between cardiovascular health and testosterone levels. Sufficient levels of testosterone may protect the cardiovascular system by assisting in blood pressure regulation and enhancing general heart health.

- Erythropoiesis: By influencing the bone marrow, testosterone promotes the synthesis of red blood cells. This process, called erythropoiesis, enhances both the blood's ability to deliver oxygen and the general health of the cardiovascular system. Strength and Muscular Development: Increasing strength and muscle development is one of testosterone's main impacts. It helps in muscle growth and repair by encouraging the production of proteins in muscle tissues. Lean body mass preservation and improved athletic performance depend on this anabolic effect.

- Bone Health: Because testosterone promotes the growth of osteoblasts, the cells that make bones, bone health is largely dependent on testosterone. Sufficient testosterone levels lower the incidence of fractures and diseases like osteoporosis by maintaining bone strength and density.
- Libido and Sexual Function: In both men and women, testosterone has a complex relationship with sexual health and function.

It affects sexual desire intensity, libido, and the general upkeep of sexual tissues. It is essential for sperm production and the healthy operation of the reproductive system in men.

- Mood and Cognitive Function: The effects of testosterone on mood and cognitive function are significant. Sufficient amounts are linked to mental clarity, optimism, and general wellbeing. Low testosterone levels have been linked in studies to irritation, mood fluctuations, and a higher chance of depression.

- Body composition and metabolism are influenced by testosterone, which also affects how energy is used and where body fat is distributed. Lean body mass is linked to optimal levels, whereas imbalances can lead to alterations in body composition, such as an increase in body fat.

- Cardiovascular Health: New research suggests a link between cardiovascular health and testosterone levels. Sufficient levels of testosterone may protect the cardiovascular system by assisting in blood pressure regulation and enhancing general heart health.

- Erythropoiesis: By influencing the bone marrow, testosterone promotes the synthesis of red blood cells. This process, called erythropoiesis, enhances both the blood's ability to deliver oxygen and the general health of the cardiovascular system.

Hormonal Regulation and Feedback Mechanisms

The endocrine system uses a complex web of feedback mechanisms to closely regulate the synthesis and release of testosterone. Gaining knowledge of these regulatory mechanisms helps one to appreciate how dynamic hormonal balance is.

- Hypothalamus-Pituitary-Gonadal (HPG) Axis: The brain region known as the hypothalamus is essential for controlling testosterone levels. It causes the pituitary gland to release luteinizing hormone (LH) and follicle-stimulating hormone by releasing gonadotropin-releasing hormone (GnRH) (FSH). Testicular Leydig cells respond specifically to LH, which initiates the production and release of testosterone.

- Negative Feedback Loop: To control its production, testosterone acts as a negative feedback loop on the HPG axis. The hypothalamus and pituitary gland are alerted to decrease the secretion of GnRH, LH, and FSH when testosterone levels rise. On the other hand, this feedback loop is lessened as testosterone levels drop, permitting more hormone synthesis and release.

- Influence of Other Hormones: Insulin and cortisol are two other hormones that have an impact on how testosterone is regulated. For instance, stress can raise cortisol levels, which may have an effect on the HPG axis and alter the way testosterone is produced. A sophisticated comprehension of these interactions is necessary to maintain hormonal homeostasis.

- Age-Related Changes: Men have a normal fall in testosterone levels as they age, a condition known as andropause. This decrease happens gradually and differs from person to person. Age-related variations in testosterone levels can affect bone density, muscle mass, and sexual function, among other aspects of health.

- Impact of External Factors: Lifestyle variables that affect testosterone levels include nutrition, exercise, and sleep patterns. Hormonal imbalances may be caused by long-term stress, insufficient sleep, and poor diet. Furthermore, the synthesis and control of testosterone may be impacted by environmental exposure to endocrine-disrupting substances. Comprehending the regulatory processes governing testosterone production illuminates the intricacy of hormonal equilibrium. The intricate interactions among the gonads, pituitary, hypothalamus, and feedback loops highlight the necessity of a comprehensive strategy for preserving ideal testosterone levels.

CHAPTER 2: SIGNS AND SYMPTOMS OF TESTOSTERONE IMBALANCE

The hormone testosterone, which plays an important role in a wide variety of physiological processes, is the subject of fine-tuning within the body. There are a variety of signs and symptoms that can be caused by an imbalance in testosterone levels, and these symptoms can have an impact on both the physical and mental health of an individual. To practice proactive health management, it is essential to recognize these indicators. In this section, we will discuss the signs and symptoms that are generally linked with testosterone imbalance. We will shed light on how these symptoms express themselves as well as the potential impact that they may have on overall good health.

Recognizing Low Testosterone Levels

- Sexual Dysfunction: Impaired sexual function is one of the main indicators of low testosterone levels. Male sexual satisfaction may decline, libido (or sex desire) may decline, and erectile dysfunction (or difficulty getting or maintaining an erection) may occur. Testosterone is essential for the upkeep of sexual tissues and the control of reproductive processes.

- Fatigue and Decreased Vitality: It is well recognized that testosterone has a role in overall vitality and energy levels. Low testosterone levels can lead to chronic weariness, low energy levels overall, and motivation deficits. This may affect day-to-day tasks, productivity at work, and tolerance to exercise.

- Loss of Strength and Muscle: Testosterone plays a major role in the growth and maintenance of muscle. Weakness and a reduction in total muscle mass might result from low testosterone levels. People could experience difficulty performing physical tasks or experience a loss of strength.

- Raised Body Fat: Testosterone regulates body composition, and low amounts are linked to an increase in body fat, especially in the abdominal region. A higher risk of metabolic problems and the emergence of central obesity may be attributed to changes in fat distribution.

- Mood swings and irritability: Testosterone affects mental health and mood. Mood fluctuations, impatience, and heightened stress susceptibility have all been associated with low testosterone levels. People can discover that they are more vulnerable to depressive or anxious thoughts.

- Sleep disturbances: The control of sleep patterns is mediated by testosterone. Low levels can be a factor in sleep disorders, insomnia, and trouble falling asleep. Sleep issues can worsen exhaustion and lower one's quality of life in general.

- Reduced Cognitive Function: Memory and focus are two areas where testosterone is involved in cognitive function. Low testosterone levels can lead to cognitive impairment, concentration problems, and a general feeling of disorientation or mental fog.

- Loss of Bone Density: Low testosterone levels can cause a reduction in bone mass because they are essential for preserving bone density. This raises the risk of fractures and osteoporosis, particularly in the elderly.

Impact on Physical and Mental Health

- Physical Health Implications: Low testosterone levels have a variety of effects on one's physical health. A sedentary lifestyle and diminished physical performance might result from reduced muscle mass and strength. Consequently, this may lead to weight increase and the emergence of diseases like diabetes and cardiovascular disease that are associated with obesity.

- Cardiovascular Health: New research indicates that low testosterone levels may be related to cardiovascular health. Unfavorable lipid profiles and high blood pressure are two cardiovascular risk factors that may arise as a result of low testosterone. Resolving the testosterone imbalance may improve heart health in general.

- Metabolic Repercussions: One of testosterone's functions in the metabolism is to control insulin sensitivity. Insulin resistance, which can hasten the onset of type 2 diabetes, is linked to low testosterone levels. For metabolic health to be maintained, hormonal balance must be maintained.

- Bone Health: Osteoporosis and fractures are more likely in postmenopausal women and older men who have reduced bone density as a result of decreased testosterone levels. This emphasizes how crucial it is to treat hormone abnormalities to maintain bone health.

- Effect on Reproductive Health: Because testosterone is necessary for the creation of sperm, low testosterone levels in men can lead to infertility. It might also have an impact on sperm motility and quality. Maintaining the health of the reproductive system requires addressing the testosterone imbalance.

- Implications for Mental Health: Testosterone has a major effect on mental health. Low testosterone levels can cause mood swings, heightened irritability, and depressive symptoms that can significantly impact a person's quality of life. Hormonal balance and mental health are linked, and treating imbalances is a necessary part of receiving complete mental health care.

- Cognitive Function: Low testosterone levels have been linked to cognitive decline, memory loss, and trouble focusing. Testosterone plays a critical role in cognitive function. Resolving hormone imbalances may help preserve mental acuity and stop age-related cognitive deterioration.

Identifying Risk Factors

- Age: One of the main risk factors for testosterone imbalance is normal aging. Age-related declines in testosterone levels are common, and people over 30 may gradually see a fall in their testosterone production. But not everyone will have noticeable symptoms, and each person's rate of decline is different.

- Obesity: Low testosterone levels are associated with obesity. Aromatase is an enzyme found in adipose tissue (fat), and it is responsible for converting testosterone into estrogen. As a result, having too much body fat can lower testosterone levels and exacerbate health problems associated with obesity.

- Chronic Illness and Medication: The production of testosterone can be impacted by some chronic illnesses, including diabetes and chronic inflammatory ailments. Furthermore, drugs like opioids and glucocorticoids may throw off the hormonal balance. People who have long-term medical illnesses should be mindful of how it can affect their testosterone levels.

- Testicular Disease or Injury: Testicular disorders or injuries can have an impact on the production of testosterone. Reduced testosterone levels can result from diseases such as testicular cancer or orchitis, an infection of the testicles.

- Hormonal Disorders: Disorders affecting the testes, pituitary gland, or hypothalamus can interfere with the hormone that regulates testosterone. Hormone imbalances can be caused by diseases including hypogonadism, pituitary tumors, and hereditary abnormalities.

- Lifestyle Factors: An imbalance in testosterone may result from several lifestyle choices. Hormone levels can be adversely affected by prolonged stress, heavy alcohol consumption, poor sleep, and a lack of physical activity. It is essential to lead a healthy lifestyle to preserve hormonal equilibrium.

- Environmental Exposures: Hormone production and regulation may be hampered by exposure to environmental variables such as endocrine-disrupting chemicals (EDCs). EDCs are present in a wide range of common products, including plastics, insecticides, and personal hygiene items.

- Genetics: Testosterone levels may also be influenced by genetic causes. Some people may be genetically predisposed to produce less testosterone, and family history may be important to take into account.

CHAPTER 3: DIAGNOSTIC APPROACHES

When it comes to preserving overall health and well-being, one of the most important aspects is recognizing and resolving any testosterone imbalance that may exist. The term "diagnostic approaches" refers to a variety of techniques that are utilized to gain an understanding of the hormonal status of an individual, evaluate symptoms, and take into consideration variables related to lifestyle. Obtaining a full grasp of hormonal health and determining testosterone levels are the primary goals of this section, in which we will discuss the most important diagnostic procedures.

Hormone Testing and Analysis

Blood Tests:

When it comes to preserving overall health and well-being, one of the most important aspects is recognizing and resolving any testosterone imbalance that may exist. The term "diagnostic approaches" refers to a variety of techniques that are utilized to gain an understanding of the hormonal status of an individual, evaluate symptoms, and take into consideration variables related to lifestyle. Obtaining a full grasp of hormonal health and determining testosterone levels are the primary goals of this section, in which we will discuss the most important diagnostic procedures.

Sex Hormone-Binding Globulin (SHBG):

There is a protein known as SHBG that can bind to sex hormones such as testosterone. It is possible to determine how much testosterone is bound and unavailable for usage by measuring the levels of SHBG. Even though total testosterone levels appear to be normal, elevated SHBG levels may be an indication of decreased bioavailable testosterone.

- **Estradiol (Estrogen) Levels:**

Measuring estrogen levels is important because testosterone can be transformed into estradiol, especially in men. Hormonal disruption symptoms can be brought on by an imbalance between estrogen and testosterone. When taking into account symptoms like gynecomastia (enlarged breast tissue) and sexual dysfunction, estradiol levels are especially important.

- **Luteinizing Hormone (LH) and Follicle-Stimulating Hormone (FSH):**

The pituitary gland secretes the hormones LH and FSH, which encourage the testes to produce more testosterone. These hormones can be measured to learn more about how the hypothalamus-pituitary-gonadal (HPG) axis is working. Low levels of LH and FSH may point to problems with the pituitary or hypothalamus, whereas high levels may indicate intrinsic testicular disease.

- **Comprehensive Hormonal Panel:**

Assessing cortisol, insulin, thyroid hormones (T3 and T4), and other hormones may be part of a full hormonal panel, including testosterone. The adoption of a more comprehensive viewpoint facilitates the assessment of endocrine health in general and aids in the identification of possible causes of hormonal imbalance.

Home Test Kits:

The creation of home test kits, which let people take blood or saliva samples at home and send them to a lab for analysis, has been made possible by advancements in healthcare technology. Although these kits can be convenient, it is important to confirm that they are accurate and reliable in comparison to standard lab-based testing.

Consultation with Healthcare Professionals

- **Endocrinologists:**

Physicians who specialize in the endocrine system, which comprises hormones and organs that produce hormones, are known as endocrinologists. Seeking advice from an endocrinologist is essential if hormonal imbalances, especially those involving testosterone, are a cause for worry. They can evaluate symptoms, decipher test results, and direct future diagnostic and therapeutic approaches.

- **Primary Care Physicians:**

A primary care physician is essential to the coordination of healthcare services. If a person exhibits symptoms indicative of a testosterone imbalance, the diagnosis can be made by their primary care physician. Initial blood tests may be ordered, symptoms may be assessed, and if necessary, the patient may be referred to an endocrinologist or other experts.

- **Urologists:**

Male reproductive organs as well as the urinary and reproductive systems are the areas of specialization for urologists. Urologists are in a good position to evaluate and treat problems relating to testosterone levels, particularly those that impact reproductive health because the testicles are the primary site of testosterone production.

- **Collaborative Care:**

Healthcare professionals frequently collaborate in their care while using diagnostic approaches. For example, to fully address hormonal and reproductive health, an endocrinologist and urologist may collaborate. A primary care physician's engagement guarantees a comprehensive approach to overall health.

Medical History and Physical Examination:

To determine potential causes of hormonal imbalances, medical experts obtain a patient's medical history and do a physical examination. During the consultation, several factors like lifestyle choices, chronic illnesses, medications, and past reproductive history are taken into account.

- **Review of Symptoms:**

We go through the symptoms of testosterone imbalance in detail, including how it affects mood, energy levels, desire, and sexual function. Healthcare providers can better comprehend a patient's subjective experiences and direct future diagnostic tests by having a thorough discussion of the symptoms.

Lifestyle and Symptom Assessment

- Lifestyle Factors: A crucial step in the diagnostic procedure is assessing lifestyle factors. Hormonal balance can be greatly impacted by lifestyle decisions about nutrition, exercise, sleep habits, and stress reduction. Healthcare providers determine whether lifestyle variables that can be changed may be a factor in testosterone imbalance and offer advice on healthy lifestyle modifications.

- Dietary Practices: Hormonal health is influenced by nutritional decisions. The best hormone production is influenced by dietary elements including getting enough calories, good fats, and all the necessary nutrients. Conversely, diets that are overly high in processed foods or deficient in essential nutrients may have a detrimental effect on hormone balance.

- Exercise and Physical Activity: Studies have demonstrated that regular exercise and physical activity raise testosterone levels. Conversely, sedentary lifestyles might be a factor in hormone abnormalities. Healthcare practitioners evaluate a person's exercise program and offer suggestions for adding physical activity to it.

- Sleep Quality: The production of testosterone and other hormones is regulated by sleep. Hormonal balance can be upset by getting too little sleep or by poor quality sleep. Medical practitioners evaluate sleep habits and may suggest methods to enhance good sleep hygiene and encourage appropriate sleep length.

- Stress management: Prolonged stress can lead to hormonal abnormalities, such as high cortisol levels, which can affect the synthesis of testosterone. A crucial part of the diagnostic process is assessing stress levels and offering advice on stress-reduction tactics including mindfulness, relaxation training, and lifestyle modifications.

- Symptom Questionnaires: A systematic evaluation of the existence and intensity of symptoms linked to a testosterone imbalance can be conducted using symptom questionnaires. Numerous topics are covered by these questionnaires, such as mood, physical well-being, energy levels, and sexual health. The findings aid medical practitioners in comprehending how symptoms affect a person's life.

- Collaboration and Patient Feedback: The diagnostic procedure depends heavily on patient feedback. A collaborative approach to care is ensured by open communication between persons experiencing symptoms of testosterone imbalance and healthcare professionals. People who actively participate in their healthcare process can offer insightful commentary on their experiences and help create individualized treatment programs.

CHAPTER 4: NUTRITION FOR TESTOSTERONE OPTIMIZATION

The process of optimizing testosterone levels is a multi-pronged activity that requires alterations to one's lifestyle, including a strategic focus on various aspects of nutrition. It is impossible to emphasize the significance of nutrition in hormonal health, as the body is dependent on a harmonious combination of macronutrients and micronutrients for the production and regulation of hormones. In the following section, we will discuss the key elements for hormonal health, identify foods that enhance testosterone levels, and detail dietary methods that support hormonal balance.

Macro and Micronutrients Essential for Hormonal Health

Protein: An essential part of any diet meant to maximize testosterone production is protein. Proteins are made up of amino acids, which are necessary for the synthesis of all hormones, including testosterone. Lean protein sources like fish, chicken, eggs, and plant-based foods like tofu and beans are good for your hormones overall.

Fats: Since hormones like testosterone are produced from cholesterol, dietary fats are essential for the generation of hormones. Hormonal balance depends on good fats, such as polyunsaturated and monounsaturated fats. Avocados, almonds, seeds, olive oil, and fatty fish high in omega-3 fatty acids are good sources of healthful fats.

Carbohydrates: A source of energy, carbohydrates affect insulin levels, which can affect the synthesis of testosterone. Eating complex carbs from fruits, vegetables, and whole grains promotes hormonal balance and helps keep blood sugar levels steady.

Vitamins: Inadequate intake of some vitamins can affect testosterone levels because they are necessary for hormonal balance. In particular, vitamin D is essential for the creation of testosterone. Vitamin D can be obtained by supplements, fortified meals, and sun exposure. Vitamins A, C, and E also maintain hormonal equilibrium indirectly and are beneficial to general health.

Minerals: Zinc and magnesium are two essential minerals for the synthesis of testosterone. Low levels of testosterone have been associated with zinc insufficiency, as zinc is a cofactor in the manufacture of testosterone. The following foods are good dietary sources of zinc: meat, seafood, nuts, and seeds. Whole grains, nuts, and leafy green vegetables are good sources of magnesium, which is needed for several metabolic functions, including hormone control.

Water: Hormonal balance and general health depend on maintaining an appropriate level of hydration. Numerous physiological systems require water, and dehydration can have a deleterious effect on hormone levels. Maintaining proper hydration promotes metabolic processes and guarantees the effective movement of nutrients necessary for hormone balance.

Testosterone-Boosting Foods

- Oysters: Oysters are a great source of zinc, which is necessary for the synthesis of testosterone. Because low testosterone levels have been linked to zinc deficiency, oysters are a great food option to promote hormonal health.

- Omega-3 fatty acids are abundant in fatty fish, including salmon, mackerel, and trout. In addition to improving general cardiovascular health, these good fats may also have a positive effect on testosterone levels.

- Eggs: Packed with healthful fats, vital amino acids, and vitamin D, eggs are a nutrient-dense food. Particularly the yolk is a source of cholesterol, which is needed for the creation of testosterone.

- Lean Meats: Lean meats, such as turkey, chicken, and lean beef cuts, are excellent sources of protein and include the vital amino acids needed to produce hormones. Including a range of lean meats contributes to a balanced diet.

- Nuts and Seeds: Rich sources of protein, healthy fats, and vital minerals like zinc and magnesium are found in nuts and seeds including almonds, walnuts, and sunflower seeds. A diverse range of nuts and seeds is a good way to support hormonal health in general.

- Avocados: High in monounsaturated fats, avocados promote healthy hormones. Avocados also include several vitamins, such as vitamin E, which is important for immune system function in general.

- Leafy Green Vegetables: High in vitamins, minerals, and antioxidants are vegetables like kale and spinach. Leafy greens include magnesium, which is necessary for several metabolic functions, including hormone regulation.

- Garlic: Allicin, a substance found in garlic, has been linked to elevated testosterone levels. Adding garlic to food improves its flavor and may have hormonal health advantages as well.

- Berries: Berries are a great source of fiber, vitamins, and antioxidants. Examples of these are blueberries and strawberries. Berries don't directly affect testosterone, but their general health benefits do assist hormonal balance in a well-rounded diet.

Dietary Strategies for Hormonal Balance

- Balanced Macronutrient Intake: For general hormonal health, it is essential to attain a balance of macronutrients, such as proteins, lipids, and carbs. Eating a diet that contains these macronutrients in the right proportions gives the body the building blocks it needs to manufacture hormones.

- Steer out of Extreme Diets: Diets that are too strict, like extremely low-carb or low-fat regimens, might throw off the hormone balance. These diets have the potential to cause dietary shortages and interfere with the complex hormonal balance. The key to nutrition is to have a sustained and balanced approach to it.

- Optimizing Vitamin D Levels: Reduced testosterone levels have been associated with vitamin D insufficiency. Maintaining ideal vitamin D levels involves getting enough sunshine, eating foods high in vitamin D, and taking supplements as needed.

- Mindful Caloric Consumption: Hormonal balance depends on maintaining a healthy weight through mindful calorie intake. Hormone control can be interfered with by both excessive body fat and severe calorie restriction. It is advised to adopt a balanced diet that promotes general well-being.

- Frequent Physical Activity: Studies have shown a correlation between increased testosterone levels and regular physical activity. Hormonal health is enhanced by strength training as well as aerobic exercise. Combining aerobic and strength training activities improves general health and hormone balance.

- Sufficient Sleep: Getting enough good sleep is crucial for controlling hormones, which includes producing testosterone. Hormonal well-being is enhanced by establishing appropriate sleep habits, aiming for 7-9 hours of sleep every night, and creating a sleep-friendly atmosphere.

- Stress management: Prolonged stress can have an adverse effect on testosterone and other hormone levels. Hormonal equilibrium is supported by incorporating stress-reduction practices like mindfulness, meditation, and relaxation exercises. Finding healthy ways to relieve stress and giving self-care a high priority are crucial elements of general well-being.

- Reducing Alcohol Intake: Studies have shown that high alcohol intake can upset the balance of hormones, particularly testosterone. It is advised to consume alcohol in moderation to promote hormonal balance and general wellness.

- Steer clear of Endocrine Disruptors: Certain plastics, insecticides, and personal hygiene items include substances known as endocrine-disrupting chemicals (EDCs), which can disrupt the balance of hormones. Choosing products free of dangerous chemicals and reducing exposure to EDCs both improve hormonal health in general.

CHAPTER 5: LIFESTYLE MODIFICATIONS

It is necessary to take a holistic strategy that goes beyond dietary considerations to achieve and maintain hormonal equilibrium. Modifications to one's lifestyle, which include engaging in regular physical activity, getting sufficient amounts of quality sleep, and effectively managing stress, are crucial in achieving optimal hormonal health. In this section, we discuss the influence that lifestyle choices have on hormonal equilibrium, with a particular emphasis on the importance of physical activity, the quality of sleep, and methods for managing stress.

Exercise and Testosterone Production

Resistance Training: Studies have shown a correlation between increased testosterone production and regular resistance or strength training workouts. Large muscular group-focused compound workouts like deadlifts and squats are especially beneficial. Growth hormones and testosterone are released in response to resistance training, which promotes muscular growth and hormonal balance in general.

High-intensity interval training, or HIIT, alternates short bursts of vigorous exercise with rest or lower-intensity activity in between. It has been demonstrated that this type of exercise improves hormonal balance, leading to higher testosterone levels. HIIT exercises save time and may be customized to meet different levels of fitness.

Aerobic Exercise: Although weight training is very beneficial, hormonal health is also enhanced by aerobic exercise. Exercises like swimming, cycling, or jogging can improve cardiovascular health and promote general well-being. A thorough fitness regimen is around striking a balance between aerobic and strength training.

Regularity and Consistency: To keep hormone balance in check, exercise regimens must be regular. Frequent exercise, whether in the form of regimented workouts or everyday mobility, promotes metabolic health and guards against hormone abnormalities, particularly those involving testosterone.

Preventing Overtraining: Although exercise is good for you, doing too much of it without enough rest periods might throw your hormones out of balance. Elevated cortisol levels from overtraining may have a detrimental effect on testosterone production. Intensity must be balanced with enough rest and recuperation time for optimal hormonal health.

Hormonal equilibrium is aided by maintaining a healthy body composition, which can be achieved by combining a balanced diet with frequent exercise. Reduced testosterone levels have been linked to excess body fat, particularly around the belly. Reaching and keeping a healthy weight promotes the best possible hormonal functioning.

Changing Up Your Exercise Routine: Including a range of exercise techniques in a regimen helps to improve hormonal balance and general fitness. A combination of resistance training, cardiovascular exercise, flexibility training, and balance and coordination-boosting activities are included in this.

Sleep Quality and Hormonal Regulation

Hormones and Circadian Rhythm: The circadian rhythm, which is the body's internal clock, is a key factor in the control of hormones. Everyday rhythms in hormone levels, such as those of melatonin and cortisol, affect sleep-wake cycles. Hormonal balance can be impacted by circadian rhythm disturbances, such as shift employment or inconsistent sleep patterns.

Production of Testosterone While Sleeping: Deep sleep, particularly in the early morning, is when testosterone is mostly generated. Maximizing testosterone levels requires undisturbed sleep for a suitable amount of time. Aiming for deep, restorative sleep cycles is vital, and people should place equal emphasis on the amount and quality of sleep.

Creating a Sleep Schedule: Maintaining a regular sleep schedule promotes hormonal balance and helps control the circadian cycle. Even on weekends, going to bed and waking up at the same time every day trains the body to expect sleep, improving the quality of sleep overall.

Sleep Hygiene Practices: Creating a sleep-friendly atmosphere starts with implementing appropriate sleep hygiene practices. This includes minimizing screen time before bed, avoiding stimulating activities right before bed, and maintaining a cold, dark, and quiet bedroom.

Reducing Alcohol and Caffeine: Both substances might impair the quality of sleep. Reducing the amount of these drugs used, particularly in the hours before bed, helps the body achieve hormonal balance and peaceful sleep.

Treating Sleep Disorders: Hormonal regulation and the quality of sleep can be adversely affected by conditions including insomnia and sleep apnea. To address underlying sleep disorders, those who are having chronic problems falling asleep should speak with healthcare specialists.

Strategic Napping: Although quick naps throughout the day can be revitalizing, taking too many or too long naps during the day can interfere with sleep patterns at night. Well-timed, quick naps can improve mental clarity without lowering the caliber of sleep at night.

Stress Management Techniques

Focusing on the current moment without passing judgment is the goal of mindfulness meditation. Reduced cortisol secretion and stress levels have been linked to regular practice. Guided imagery, body scan meditations, and focused breathing are examples of mindfulness practices.

Exercises for Deep Breathing: Deep breathing techniques, such as diaphragmatic or belly breathing, cause the body to go into relaxation mode. Regular use of these strategies can help to lower cortisol levels, alleviate stress, and foster a sense of calm.

Yoga and Tai Chi: Mind-body exercises that combine breathing, movement, and mindfulness are yoga and tai chi. Research indicates that engaging in these activities might lower stress and improve general well-being. These exercises' soft, flowing motions might be especially helpful for stress relief.

Frequent Exercise: Exercise has major favorable effects on mental health in addition to its physical benefits. The body's natural mood enhancers, endorphins, are released when you exercise, and this can help reduce the symptoms of stress and anxiety.

Time management: Setting realistic objectives and using your time wisely might help you feel less stressed and overwhelmed. Reducing stress can be achieved by prioritizing work, breaking it down into manageable chunks, and scheduling downtime for self-care and relaxation.

Social Support: Retaining social ties and asking friends, family, or support groups for assistance can be very helpful in stress management. Emotional well-being is influenced by talking about worries, getting counsel, and encouraging healthy social relationships.

Holistic Methods: Acupuncture, massage therapy, aromatherapy, and other holistic methods of stress reduction can be used in addition to lifestyle changes. These methods encourage relaxation and could enhance general well-being.

Setting Limits: Clearly defining boundaries in both personal and professional spheres aids with stress management. Setting limits includes knowing when to say no, emphasizing self-care, and identifying situations in which taking on more obligations could cause unnecessary stress.

CHAPTER 6: SUPPLEMENTS AND HERBS FOR TESTOSTERONE SUPPORT

Modifications to one's lifestyle, dietary decisions, and, in some instances, supplementation with herbs and particular nutrients are all components of the multidimensional strategy that is required to achieve optimal testosterone levels. This section provides an introduction to testosterone-boosting supplements, investigates herbal therapies that are supported by data, and discusses the dose and safety considerations involved in using these supplements.

Overview of Testosterone-Boosting Supplements

1. Deficit in vitamin D has been linked to reduced levels of testosterone, which is a consequence of the fact that vitamin D is essential for the production of testosterone. Sunlight exposure, dietary sources, and supplementation are all viable options for achieving and maintaining adequate levels of vitamin D. For each individual, the dosage should be tailored to their specific requirements and levels.

2. Zinc: Zinc is an essential mineral that plays a role in the creation of testosterone. In the process of hormone manufacturing, it performs the function of a cofactor. Even

though zinc shortage might result in decreased testosterone levels, it is important to avoid taking an excessive amount of supplements. The amount of zinc that is recommended to be consumed daily varies, and it is vital to find a balance to achieve optimal hormonal health.

3. Magnesium: Magnesium is involved in several metabolic processes, including those that are associated with the regulation of hormone activities. Magnesium supplementation may have a beneficial effect on testosterone levels, particularly in persons who are struggling with shortages, according to the findings of several studies.

Depending on the individual's needs and current state of health, dosage recommendations are made.

4. Fish Oil Supplements Omega-3 Fatty Acids Omega-3 fatty acids, which can be found in fatty fish and fish oil supplements, can reduce inflammation and may also help the general health of the hormones. Omega-3 fatty acid supplementation is beneficial for cardiovascular health and may indirectly improve hormonal balance. Although limited data indicates direct testosterone-boosting effects, omega-3 supplementation is beneficial for prostate health.

5. D-Aspartic Acid (DAA): DAA is an amino acid that is involved in the production of testosterone as well as its release. Some studies suggest that taking DAA supplements could result in higher levels of testosterone, particularly in people who had low levels of testosterone at the beginning of the study. On the other hand, additional research is required to determine the efficacy and safety over the long run.

6. The herb known as fenugreek has a long history of use in cultures around the world for its ability to boost libido and masculinity. The addition of fenugreek may have a beneficial effect on testosterone levels, according to the findings of several studies.

A number of different preparations, including teas and supplements, are available for purchase.

7. Tribulus Terrestris: Tribulus terrestris is a herb that has been sold as a testosterone enhancer through several marketing channels. There is little data to support the claim that it is beneficial in raising testosterone levels, even though certain research has suggested that it may have potential benefits for libido and sexual function.

8. Ashwagandha: Ashwagandha is a herb that can reduce stress and is considered an adaptogenic herb. According to the findings

of a few research, using ashwagandha supplements may result in higher levels of testosterone and enhanced reproductive health. The recommended dosage can change depending on the particular product.

Evidence-Based Herbal Remedies

- Tongkat Ali, also known as Eurycoma Longifolia, is a herb that has long been used to increase libido and male fertility. It may raise testosterone levels, according to some studies, but further research is required to confirm its safety and effectiveness.

- Ginseng: Research has been conducted on the possible support of testosterone with ginseng, namely Panax ginseng. Although studies are still being conducted, some point to the potential benefits of ginseng for testosterone levels and male reproductive health.

- Maca Root: Traditionally utilized for its possible aphrodisiac properties, maca root is a native of Peru. Supplementing with maca may boost libido and enhance semen quality, according to certain research. More research is needed to determine how it affects testosterone levels.

- Nettle Root: The possibility that nettle root may help raise free testosterone levels by preventing testosterone from attaching to sex hormone-binding globulin (SHBG) has been investigated. To determine the best dosage and level of effectiveness, more study is required.

- Pine Bark Extract (Pycnogenol): Packed with antioxidants, Pycnogenol, also known as pine bark extract, has been researched for several health advantages. Although further research is required to validate its efficacy and safety, some evidence points to possible good benefits on testosterone levels.

- Rhodiola rosea: This adaptogenic plant may aid the body in adjusting to stressful situations. It is well known for its ability to alleviate hormone imbalances brought on by stress, even though there is little study on how it affects testosterone.

- Saw Palmetto: Studies have indicated that saw palmetto, which is frequently used to support prostate health, may have a slight effect on testosterone levels. It is frequently present in supplements meant to promote the health of male reproduction.

Dosage and Safety Considerations

- Individual Variability: Age, health, and pre-existing illnesses are just a few examples of individual characteristics that can affect the dosage recommendations for vitamins and herbs. A healthcare provider should be consulted to determine the proper dosages based on each person's needs.

- Monitoring Hormone Levels: When thinking about supplements, it's important to regularly evaluate hormonal levels. This helps avoid any imbalances or negative effects and permits dosage modifications based on individual reactions.

- Consultation with Healthcare Specialists: It is imperative to get advice from healthcare professionals, especially those with endocrinology expertise, before beginning any supplement plan. They can evaluate each person's health status, offer advice on appropriate dosages, and keep an eye out for any possible drug interactions or pre-existing diseases.

- Supplement Quality: The purity and quality of supplements are very important. Selecting reliable brands and goods that go through independent testing to check their quality and potency guarantees that people get the benefits they need without coming into contact with harmful substances.

- Possible Interactions: Certain drugs or pre-existing medical conditions may interact with certain vitamins and herbs. To evaluate possible interactions and prevent negative effects, it is essential to report to healthcare providers any medications and supplements being taken.

- Length of Supplementation: Depending on personal requirements and objectives, the length of supplementation may differ. Long-term use for maintaining general health may not be the same as short-term use for particular goals, including correcting deficits. Healthcare experts can offer advice on suitable times.

- Safety of Herbal Remedies: Although many herbs have been traditionally utilized for a range of health advantages, there may be differences in their safety profiles. Certain plants may interact with drugs or have unintended effects. People should use caution, especially if they are pregnant or have a history of medical issues.

- Lifestyle Factors: The best results from supplements and herbs come from a comprehensive strategy that incorporates lifestyle changes. All of these factors—diet, exercise, restful sleep, and stress reduction—have an impact on hormone balance overall.

CHAPTER 7: HORMONE REPLACEMENT THERAPY (HRT)

Hormone Replacement Therapy, also known as HRT, is a medical intervention that is aimed at alleviating hormonal imbalances by supplementing or replacing hormones that are lacking in the treatment. It is normal practice to use hormone replacement therapy (HRT) in the context of testosterone to treat diseases that are associated with low testosterone levels, which is a condition known as hypogonadism. In this section, we go into the complexities of hormone replacement therapy, discussing its history, the many methods of testosterone replacement, as well as the dangers, benefits, and considerations that are connected with it.

Introduction to HRT

Essential messengers and hormones control many bodily physiological functions. When there is an imbalance, people may experience symptoms including weariness, poor libido, mood swings, and decreased muscle mass, depending on the cause—aging, medical disorders, or other causes. The goals of hormone replacement therapy are to promote general health, relieve symptoms, and restore hormonal balance.

- Testosterone replacement therapy is indicated when necessary since it plays several roles in male sex development, maintenance of bone density, muscle mass, and libido, among other things. Insufficient production of testosterone, or hypogonadism, can be caused by aging, certain drugs, or medical diseases such as pituitary malfunction or disorders of the testicles.

- Forms of HRT: There are several ways to deliver HRT, such as injections, gels, patches, and pellets. The mode of administration chosen will rely on personal preferences, health issues, and advice from the healthcare professional.

- Advantages of Testosterone Replacement Therapy: The advantages of testosterone replacement therapy go beyond curing particular ailments. It might provide greater energy, a happier mood, more muscular growth, and stronger bones. Additionally, for those suffering from the symptoms of low testosterone, HRT can improve general quality of life and sexual performance.

- Customized Treatment Plans: There is no one-size-fits-all method when it comes to HRT. Healthcare professionals develop individualized treatment programs by evaluating each patient's health status, symptoms, and medical history. Frequent monitoring reduces the possibility of side effects by ensuring that hormone levels are within an ideal range.

Types of Testosterone Replacement

- Direct injections of testosterone into the muscles are known as intramuscular injections. With this approach, the hormone can be released gradually into the bloodstream; normally, injections are needed every one to two weeks. Testosterone enanthate and testosterone cypionate are common formulations.

- Topical Gels and Patches: Transdermal testosterone administration is offered by topical formulations like gels and patches. While patches stick to the skin and gradually release testosterone, gels are administered to the skin, usually on the shoulders, upper arms, or abdomen. People who want noninvasive methods may prefer this one since it maintains stable hormone levels.

- Testosterone pellets, also known as implantable subcutaneous devices, are tiny devices that are placed under the skin and release a consistent amount of testosterone over months. This approach is convenient because it does not require repeated administrations. The effects of pellets, which are usually injected beneath the skin, can extend for three to six months.

- Oral Tablets: There are oral testosterone tablets available, albeit they are less prevalent. However, because of worries regarding their safety profile and their propensity for liver damage, they are not as frequently given.

Risks, Benefits, and Considerations

- **Benefits of Testosterone Replacement:**
  - Better Quality of Life: By treating low testosterone symptoms including exhaustion, mood swings, and decreased libido, hormone replacement therapy (HRT) can improve general well-being.
  - Bone Density and Muscle Mass: The preservation of bone density and muscle mass depends on testosterone. By improving bone density and muscle strength, HRT can lower the risk of fractures.
- **Risks and Considerations:**
  - Risk of Cardiovascular Events: Studies have indicated a possible link between testosterone replacement therapy and a higher chance of cardiovascular events.

Nonetheless, the data is still unclear, so medical professionals carefully consider cardiovascular risk factors before recommending hormone replacement therapy.

- Prostate Health: The effect of testosterone replacement therapy on prostate health is a topic of continuous discussion. Although there have been some worries expressed regarding a possible connection to prostate cancer, the available data does not support a firm association. Prostate monitoring regularly is crucial for people using HRT.

- Erythrocytosis (Increased Red Blood Cell Count): Red blood cell synthesis can be stimulated by testosterone replacement.

Despite being generally well-tolerated, this side effect has the potential to cause erythrocytosis, a disorder marked by an increased red blood cell count. This possible side effect is better managed with routine blood monitoring.

- **Individualized Treatment Plans and Monitoring:**
  - Baseline Assessment: To establish baseline values, healthcare providers do a comprehensive assessment, which includes a review of medical history, physical examination, and hormonal testing, before starting hormone replacement therapy (HRT).

- Frequent Monitoring: To modify treatment regimens and handle any possible adverse effects, ongoing monitoring is essential. Regular blood tests measure hematocrit, hormone levels, and other pertinent variables.

- Customized Doses: Doses are adjusted based on each person's requirements and reaction. Based on hormone levels, the remission of symptoms, and any possible adverse effects, adjustments may be made.

- **Potential Side Effects:**

  - Skin Reactions and Acne: When topical formulations are applied, skin reactions such as acne or irritation may develop.

- Fluid Retention: Swelling may result from fluid retention in certain people.

- Mood swings: In certain situations, mood swings, increased hostility, or impatience may manifest.

- **Long-Term Considerations:**

- Bone Health: Testosterone contributes to the preservation of bone mass. Osteoporosis risk can be decreased and bone health can be enhanced with long-term hormone replacement therapy.

- Age-Related Changes: To account for shifting hormonal requirements, people of a certain age may require modifications to the frequency and dosage of testosterone replacement therapy.

- **Cautions for Specific Populations:**

    - Pediatric and Teenage Considerations: In cases of delayed puberty or certain medical disorders, testosterone replacement therapy is usually reserved for pediatric and adolescent populations, requiring special consideration.

    - Pregnancy and Breastfeeding: It is not recommended to replace testosterone while pregnant or nursing. For a newborn or developing fetus, it may have masculinizing effects.

CHAPTER 8: NATURAL APPROACHES TO TESTOSTERONE ENHANCEMENT

It is possible to achieve and maintain adequate testosterone levels through the use of natural, holistic methods that emphasize lifestyle, mind-body activities, and environmental influences. In this section, we will discuss natural methods for increasing testosterone levels. These methods include mind-body activities, taking into account environmental influences, and holistic approaches to hormonal health.

Mind-Body Practices

Stress Reduction through Mindfulness:

A decrease in testosterone levels is one of the contributing factors that might lead to hormonal abnormalities brought on by chronic stress. Through the activation of the body's relaxation response, mindfulness activities, such as meditation and exercises that include deep breathing, are beneficial in the management of stress. Regular practice of mindfulness has been linked to lower levels of the stress hormone cortisol, which in turn promotes increased hormonal equilibrium.

- **Good Sleep and Circadian Rhythms:** Deep sleep is when testosterone production is most active, and sleep is essential for maintaining hormonal balance. Hormonal balance is influenced by establishing regular sleep schedules, giving priority to a sleep-friendly environment, and making sure you get 7-9 hours of good sleep every night. Syncing with circadian rhythms promotes general health.

- **Exercise and Testosterone:** Studies have shown a correlation between elevated testosterone levels and regular physical activity, which includes both resistance training and aerobic exercise. Exercises like deadlifts and squats that concentrate on large muscular groups can be very beneficial. Maintaining a healthy balance between the various types of exercise promotes hormonal balance and general fitness.

- **Hormones and Weight Management:** Hormone balance depends on maintaining a healthy weight. Reduced testosterone levels are linked to excess body fat, particularly around the belly. Maintaining hormonal balance and managing weight is enhanced by eating a balanced diet and doing frequent exercise.

- **Intimacy and Sexual Activity:** Having intimate relationships and engaging in sexual activity can raise testosterone levels. In addition to enhancing general well-being, healthy sexual engagement can help maintain hormonal balance. Sustaining hormonal health naturally includes maintaining a fulfilling and satisfied sexual life.

- **Emotional Health and Social Connectivity:** Developing and sustaining social ties has a beneficial effect on emotional health, which in turn supports hormonal balance. A feeling of purpose, emotional support, and meaningful relationships are essential elements of holistic wellness.

Environmental Factors and Endocrine Disruptors

Avoiding Endocrine Disruptors:

Substances that interfere with the hormone system are known as endocrine disruptors. Endocrine disruptors include some of the compounds in plastics, insecticides, and several personal hygiene items. Reducing exposure to these drugs supports healthy hormones.

Choosing Natural and Organic Products:

Choosing natural and organic products minimizes exposure to potentially hazardous chemicals. Examples of such products include cleaning supplies and personal care items. A more hormonally friendly environment is supported by reading labels, purchasing organic products, and avoiding endocrine-disrupting chemicals in items.

Balancing Hormones with Nutrition:

There are natural substances in some foods that could aid with hormone balance. As an illustration:

- **Cruciferous Vegetables:** Indole-3-carbinol, found in broccoli, cauliflower, and Brussels sprouts, may help support the metabolism of estrogens.

- **Flaxseeds:** Flaxseeds, being high in lignans, might have a slight estrogenic impact.

- **Zinc-Rich Foods:** Zinc, which is present in foods like oysters, almonds, and seeds, is necessary for the synthesis of testosterone.

- **Fiber-Rich Foods:** A high-fiber diet promotes gut health, which is connected to the balance of hormones in the body.

Hydration and Detoxification:

To promote the natural detoxification processes of the body, staying hydrated is essential. In addition to assisting in the elimination of pollutants and promoting general metabolic health, drinking a proper amount of water also serves to contribute to hormonal equilibrium.

Holistic Approaches to Hormonal Health

Herbal Supplements and Adaptogens:

Hormone health has traditionally been supported by the use of certain herbs and adaptogens. For example, consider:

- **Ashwagandha:** An adaptogenic plant that could aid in cortisol regulation and stress management.
- **Rhodiola Rosea:** An additional adaptogen that may have anti-stress properties.
- **Maca Root:** renowned for its ability to enhance sexual function and libido.

Balanced Nutrition for Hormonal Health:

For hormonal health, it is essential to choose a diet rich in nutrients and well-balanced. Important nutrients consist of:

- **Omega-3 Fatty Acids:** Omega-3 fatty acids, which are present in walnuts, flaxseeds, and fatty fish, are good for your general health and may even balance hormones.

- **Vitamin D:** Vitamin D is received by sunlight exposure, food sources, and supplements if needed. It is essential for the synthesis of testosterone.

- **Protein and Healthy Fats:** Hormone production and general well-being are enhanced by eating enough protein and healthy fats like avocados and olive oil.

Intermittent Fasting:

The possible effects of intermittent fasting, which alternates between eating and fasting intervals, have been investigated concerning hormone health. Intermittent fasting has been linked to improved testosterone levels and metabolic health, according to some studies.

Limiting Alcohol and Caffeine:

Overindulgence in alcohol can have a deleterious effect on the balance of hormones, particularly testosterone. In a similar vein, excessive coffee consumption can cause stress and interfere with sleep, which might affect hormonal balance. Consuming alcohol and caffeine in moderation promotes general well-being.

Mind-Body Practices for Stress Management:

Stress can be managed by incorporating mind-body exercises like tai chi, yoga, and meditation into everyday routines. Hormonal imbalances can be caused by prolonged stress, and these techniques offer strategies for mental and physical well-being.

Limiting Exposure to Blue Light:

Sleep patterns and circadian cycles can be upset and sleep-related issues might arise from exposure to artificial light, particularly blue light from screens. Adopting exposure-limiting techniques, including wearing blue light filters at night, promotes hormonal equilibrium and the body's natural sleep-wake cycles.

Regular Health Checkups:

Frequent examinations offer the chance to evaluate hormonal balance and track general health. If hormone abnormalities are found, medical professionals can measure hormone levels and offer advice on changing one's lifestyle.

CHAPTER 9: CASE STUDIES

To gain significant insights into the issues that individuals confront when navigating hormonal health, the solutions that they adopt, and the lessons that they learn along the road, it is important to have an understanding of the real-life experiences of individuals. In this part of the article, we will examine case studies that shed light on the various endeavors that individuals undertake to achieve hormonal equilibrium.

Real-Life Experiences and Success Stories

John's Journey to Hormonal Balance:

Context: John, a 45-year-old CEO, started to exhibit signs of low testosterone, such as mood swings, decreased libido, and exhaustion. He sought the advice of a healthcare expert to take a comprehensive strategy.

Interventions:

Lifestyle Modification: John undertook a thorough lifestyle makeover that included consistent exercise, better eating habits, and stress reduction techniques.

Testosterone Replacement Therapy (TRT): To address John's hormonal imbalance, his healthcare practitioner came up with a customized TRT plan that included testosterone injections after a thorough assessment.

Outcomes:

Resolution of Symptoms: John's symptoms gradually improved over time, showing signs of renewed libido, improved mood, and higher vitality.

Lifestyle Integration: John did not alter his way of living; he still placed a strong emphasis on the value of regular exercise, a balanced diet, and mindfulness exercises.

Sarah's Hormonal Health During Menopause:

Background: Hot flashes, mood swings, and disturbed sleep were just a few of the symptoms that 52-year-old Sarah experienced as she approached menopause. In search of a more natural solution, she sought advice from a holistic medical professional.

Interventions:

Nutritional Advice: Sarah was given individualized advice on how to incorporate foods that support hormones, such as leafy greens and flaxseeds, into her diet.

Herbal Pills: To aid with menopausal symptoms, her doctor suggested herbal supplements including dong quai and black cohosh.

Mind-Body Techniques: Sarah adopted yoga and mindfulness meditation as a way to reduce stress and enhance her general well-being.

Outcomes:

Symptom Relief: Sarah saw a decrease in the frequency and severity of her mood swings and hot flashes.

Improvement in Quality of Life: During the menopausal transition, a combination of mind-body techniques, herbal supplements, and proper nutrition led to an improvement in quality of life.

Challenges and Solutions

James' Struggle with Stress-Related Hormonal Imbalances:

Challenge: James, a 38-year-old professional, had persistent stress as a result of his demanding personal and professional obligations, which resulted in symptoms including low energy, weight gain, and insomnia.

Solution:

Stress Reduction Strategies: James implemented regular breaks from work and mindfulness meditation as well as other everyday stress reduction strategies.

Frequent Exercise: James found that regular physical activity, especially aerobic exercise, helped him manage his stress and maintain his hormone balance overall.

Outcome:

Stress Reduction: Regular exercise and the application of stress management techniques led to a discernible decrease in stress levels. James reported feeling more energized and having better quality sleep.

Amy's Post-Pregnancy Hormonal Status:

Challenge: Amy, a 30-year-old new mother, had mood swings, exhaustion, and irregular sleep patterns as a result of hormonal changes she had after giving birth.

Solution:

Balanced Nutrition: Amy concentrated on eating a diet high in nutrients, such as foods high in iron, vitamins, and omega-3 fatty acids, which are essential for postpartum healing and hormone balance.

Postpartum Support Group: Amy was able to get emotional support and a forum to talk with other mothers about her experiences by joining a postpartum support group.

Outcome:

Progressive Reduction in Symptoms: Although hormonal swings are typical after childbirth, Amy's dedication to a healthy diet and mental health, together with the support of the postpartum community, helped her symptoms gradually become better.

Lessons Learned

Customized Strategies Are Essential:

Lesson: The case studies emphasize how crucial it is to customize interventions to meet the needs of each individual. There isn't one answer that works for everyone, and medical professionals are essential in identifying and addressing each person's specific needs.

A Key Role for Lifestyle: Lesson Nutrition, exercise, and stress reduction are among the lifestyle changes that are regularly identified as essential to establishing hormonal balance. Long-term well-being is facilitated by long-term, sustainable adjustments in daily routines.

Holistic health is a multifaceted concept that includes mental, emotional, and physical well-being, among other things. A holistic approach to hormonal health combines mind-body practices, nutritional techniques, and, where needed, medical therapies.

Lesson: Stress Management Is Not Negotiable Hormonal abnormalities are often caused by prolonged stress. Not only are stress management practices like regular exercise and mindfulness useful for overall mental and emotional well-being, but they are also beneficial for hormonal health.

Frequent observation is crucial.

Lesson: It is essential to continuously assess hormone levels, symptoms, and general health. Visits with medical professionals regularly enable treatment plans to be modified, guaranteeing that interventions stay efficient and in line with patient requirements.

Social and Emotional Support Are Important: Lesson Participating in support groups offers a feeling of community and emotional support, whether the group is for new moms or people with comparable health issues. During health journeys, it can be empowering to share experiences and learn from others.

Lesson: Patient education empowers People can take an active role in their health by learning about the complexities of hormonal health. Making well-informed decisions is enhanced when one is aware of the effects of lifestyle decisions and the functions of different interventions.

CHAPTER 10: FUTURE TRENDS AND EMERGING RESEARCH

Throughout the ongoing development of the field of hormonal health, researchers and professionals working in the healthcare industry are investigating novel approaches, carrying out ongoing studies, and looking for breakthroughs that could have a significant impact on the future of hormonal therapy. This section delves into the most recent developments and developing research in the field of hormonal health, with a particular emphasis on the latest advancements, ongoing studies, and the ever-changing environment of testosterone therapy research.

- **Precision Medicine and Personalized Hormonal Therapies:** New Frontiers in Healthcare Genetic research and precision medicine advancements are opening the path for individualized hormone therapy. Individualizing interventions based on genetic makeup and hormone profiles allows for more targeted and successful treatments.

- **Innovation in Telemedicine and Hormonal Health:** Telemedicine incorporation with hormonal health practices increases access to specialist care. Individuals can receive hormonal health support from the comfort of their own homes thanks to virtual consultations, remote monitoring, and digital health platforms.

- **Innovation in Hormonal Health Management Using Artificial Intelligence (AI):** Artificial intelligence is increasingly being used to examine massive datasets and detect patterns in hormonal health. Individual reactions can help machine learning algorithms forecast hormone imbalances, optimize treatment strategies, and personalize remedies.

- **Innovation in Bioidentical Hormones and Novel Delivery Systems:** Bioidentical hormones, which replicate the chemical structure of hormones produced naturally in the body, are gaining popularity. Transdermal patches, subcutaneous implants, and tailored formulations are examples of novel delivery systems that attempt to improve the efficacy and safety of hormone therapy.

Ongoing Studies and Potential Breakthroughs

Gut Microbiota and Hormonal Function: A Current Research Focus The body of research examining the relationship between hormone balance and gut bacteria is growing. Novel treatments for hormonal abnormalities may result from our growing understanding of how the microbiota affects hormone synthesis and metabolism.

Current Research on Hormonal Regulation and Epigenetics Studies on epigenetics look into how the environment affects hormone regulation and gene expression. Understanding epigenetic pathways may open up new therapeutic avenues for treating imbalances and maintaining hormonal health.

Peptide Treatments and Hormone Control: Current Research The use of tiny proteins in peptide treatments is being investigated for its ability to control hormones. Peptides' potential to improve hormonal function, and balance, and treat particular hormonal deficits is being investigated.

Current Research on Hormonal Optimization and Circadian Rhythms Research into the complex link between hormone variations and circadian rhythms is still ongoing. Understanding how hormone release is regulated by the circadian rhythm may enable more effective therapies for hormonal wellness.

- **Non-Hormonal Methods for Endocrine Health:**

  Possible Pioneers: Non-hormonal strategies, such as new drugs and treatments that focus on pathways connected to hormonal balance, are being researched. These strategies seek to offer less potentially harmful substitutes for conventional hormone therapies.

The Evolving Landscape of Testosterone Therapy

Extended-Duration Testosterone Supplements:

Innovation: The goal of long-acting testosterone formulations, including injectables with extended-release characteristics, is to lessen how often the medication must be administered. These combinations are practical and could improve patient compliance.

Innovations for Topical and Transdermal Applications: Enhancements in testosterone formulations for topical and transdermal applications encompass enhanced absorption technologies and optimized delivery methods. These developments are intended to increase effectiveness while reducing the possibility of skin irritation linked to specific formulations.

Research on SARMs (Selective Androgen Receptor Modulators): Current Studies Selective androgen receptor modulators, or SARMs, may offer advantages comparable to those of testosterone but with fewer adverse effects. The effectiveness and safety of SARMs for testosterone optimization are still being investigated.

Hormonal Synergy and Combination Therapies: Innovation To produce synergistic effects, researchers are investigating the possible advantages of combining testosterone with other hormones or treatments. Combining treatments can improve results while reducing negative effects brought on by increased dosages of individual hormones.

Innovative Digital Health Platforms for Testosterone Management: Platforms for digital health are being created to assist those receiving testosterone therapy. To improve patient involvement and adherence, these systems might have features like virtual consultations, symptom tracking, and prescription reminders.

Current Research on Preserving Fertility During Testosterone Therapy Since testosterone treatment can affect fertility, research is currently being done to find ways to preserve fertility in those receiving testosterone treatment. Investigating the use of gonadotropin-releasing hormone agonists to sustain sperm production is one aspect of this.

Age-Optimized Prescription of Testosterone: New Approach: More focus is being placed on age-specific testosterone therapy demands. Age-optimized prescribing provides individualized treatment programs by taking into account changes in hormone levels, metabolism, and general health as people age.

CONCLUSION

Throughout this in-depth investigation of testosterone-building therapy, we have traversed the complexities of hormonal health, beginning with an understanding of the significance of testosterone and progressing to the investigation of diagnostic methods, lifestyle adjustments, and cutting-edge research. As we come to a close, let us review the most important points, encourage readers to take charge of their hormonal health, and share some concluding ideas and words of encouragement for living a life that is both balanced and successful.

Recap of Key Takeaways

A vital hormone balance is:

Comprehending the significance of hormonal equilibrium, specifically testosterone, is fundamental to general health and wellness. Hormones are essential for many physiological functions; they affect mood, sexual function, energy levels, and more.

Numerous Factors Affect Hormonal Health: Numerous factors, such as age, heredity, lifestyle, and exposure to the environment, can affect one's hormonal health. An all-encompassing strategy for hormonal well-being is made possible by the realization of how these variables are interrelated.

Understanding the Signs of Imbalance is Essential:

Early intervention requires an awareness of the warning signs and symptoms of hormone imbalance. Fatigue, mood swings, poor libido, and irregular sleep patterns are examples of symptoms that could point to hormonal problems that need to be addressed.

All-inclusive Diagnostic Methods are accessible:

A thorough awareness of hormonal state is provided by diagnostic techniques, which include hormone testing, professional consultation, lifestyle and symptom assessments, and consultation with medical professionals. A precise diagnosis provides the groundwork for customized interventions.

Lifestyle and Nutrition Have a Big Impact:

Modifications to lifestyle, exercise, and nutrition are effective strategies for enhancing hormonal health. An atmosphere that is hormone-friendly is enhanced by nutrient-dense foods, frequent exercise, and stress management.

The Role of Therapies and Supplements:

Depending on a patient's needs and under the supervision of medical specialists, targeted supplements, herbal therapies, and hormone replacement therapy (HRT) may be taken into consideration. These therapies seek to improve general well-being by addressing certain imbalances.

Natural Methods Support Conventional Therapies:

Holistic methods, environmental factors, and mind-body techniques offer supplementary ways to promote hormonal balance. These organic methods support a sustainable and well-balanced way of life.

Future Research Shapes It: New developments, continuing research, and a changing field for testosterone therapy will define the future of hormonal health. Our understanding of hormonal well-being is being shaped by advances in artificial intelligence, telemedicine, precision medicine, and gut microbiome research.

Final Thoughts and Encouragement

Starting a path to achieve optimal hormonal health is a commitment to living a healthy, satisfying life. Here are some closing ideas and motivational statements before we wrap up:

Understanding that hormonal health is a lifelong process that changes with age and situational changes is important. Accept the trip with an open mind, flexibility, and dedication to your continued well-being.

Honor Development Rather Than Perfection:

Consistent efforts lead to a cumulative improvement in hormonal health. Honor modest accomplishments, constructive lifestyle adjustments, and the body's resiliency. Make progress your priority instead of perfection.

Seek Advice and Assistance: Don't be afraid to ask dietitians, mental health specialists, and medical professionals for advice and support. Creating a network of support and asking for help when you need it are crucial elements of a holistic approach to health.

Put Self-Care First: Taking care of oneself is essential for hormonal balance, not a luxury. Make self-care activities that make you happy, calm, and refreshed a priority. Make self-care an indispensable part of your routine, whether it takes the form of a warm bath, a leisurely walk, or quality time with loved ones.

Accept the Wisdom of Balance: The fundamental idea behind hormonal health is balance. The body achieves balance when work and rest, diet and indulgence, and exercise and leisure are all balanced. Accept the principle of harmony in all facets of your existence.

Have faith in the body's intrinsic wisdom: the body knows how to keep itself in balance and good health. Have faith in the body's capacity to heal, adapt, and prosper. You may help the body's natural functions by adopting lifestyle choices that provide the ideal environment.

Celebrate Your Health Journey: Every person's health journey is different, containing learning experiences, obstacles, and growth opportunities. Recognize the work you put into your well-being and enjoy the ride. You become healthier and more energetic with every step you take.